ANXIE

50 HABITS TO OVERCOME & PREVENT ANXIETY AND DEPRESSION

*Self-Therapy & Cognitive Behavioral Therapy
Positive Mind & Mood Using Affirmations Self-Love
& Set Boundaries*

DR. R. AHMED

Copyrights and Trademarks

© Copyright 2023 Dr. R. Ahmed, Book Passion LLC – All rights reserved

All rights reserved. No part of this book may be reproduced or transformed in any form or by any means, graphic, electronic, or mechanical, including photocopying, recording, taping, or by any information storage retrieval system, without the author's written permission.

ISBN: 979-8-9878572-4-3

DEDICATION

This book is dedicated to all those who suffer from, treat, and care about mental health diseases, especially anxiety and depression.

DISCLAIMER

This book details the author's personal experiences with and opinions about managing anxiety and depression. The author is not your healthcare provider.

The author and publisher are providing this book and its contents on an "as is" basis and make no representations or warranties of any kind with respect to this book or its contents. The author and publisher disclaim all such representations and warranties, including for example warranties of merchantability and healthcare for a particular purpose. In addition, the author and publisher do not represent or warrant that the information accessible via this book is accurate, complete or current.

The statements made about products and services have not been evaluated by the U.S. Food and Drug Administration. They are not intended to diagnose, treat, cure, or prevent any condition or disease. Please consult with your own physician or healthcare specialist regarding the suggestions and recommendations made in this book.

Except as specifically stated in this book, neither the author or publisher, nor any authors, contributors, or other representatives will be liable for damages arising out of or in connection with the use of this book.

This is a comprehensive limitation of liability that applies to all damages of any kind, including (without limitation) compensatory; direct, indirect or consequential damages; loss of data, income or profit; loss of or damage to property and claims of third parties.

You understand that this book is not intended as a substitute for consultation with a licensed healthcare practitioner, such as your physician. Before you begin any healthcare program, or change your lifestyle in any way, you will consult your physician or another licensed healthcare practitioner to ensure that you are in good health and that the examples contained in this book will not harm you.

This book provides content related to physical and/or mental health issues. As such, use of this book implies your acceptance of this disclaimer.

TABLE OF CONTENTS

ACKNOWLEDGMENTS 1
1 - EXERCISE 3
2 – SPEND TIME OUTDOORS 7
3 - MINDFULNESS 9
4 - COGNITIVE BEHAVIORAL THERAPY 11
5 – JOIN A SUPPORT GROUP 13
6 - JOURNAL 15
7 – PAINTING, DRAWING, COLORING 17
8 - MUSIC 19
9 – FUN ACTIVITIES 21
10 – CONNECT WITH A PERSON YOU TRUST 23
11 – SEEK COUNSELING 25
12 – DEEP BREATHING EXERCISES 27
13 – SET GOALS 29
14 – SLEEP WELL 32
15 – YOGA 34
16 – VOLUNTEER 36
17 – AROMATHERAPY 38
18 – STAY AWAY FROM DRUGS 40
19 – BALANCED DIET & STAY HYDRATED 42
20 – TOXIC PEOPLE & TOXIC FAMILY 46
21 – CUT CAFFEINE 50

22 – LIMIT ALCOHOL	52
23 – LIMIT TIME ON SOCIAL MEDIA	54
24 – PRACTICE SELF-CARE	56
25 – TAKE A BATH	58
26 – POSITIVE AFFIRMATIONS	60
27 – BE ORGANIZED	62
28 – DAILY ROUTINE	64
29 – TREAT UNDERLYING MEDICAL CONDITIONS	66
30 – LIMIT NEGATIVE NEWS OR MEDIA	68
31 – PRACTICE GRATITUDE	70
32 – POSITIVE PEOPLE	72
33 – HOBBIES	74
34 – LEARN A NEW SKILL	76
35 – HEALTHY THYROID	78
36 – FORGIVE YOURSELF & OTHERS	80
37 – AVOID ISOLATION	82
38 – SET BOUNDARIES	84
39 – LEARN TO SAY NO	86
40 – MEDITATE	88
41 – PRAY	90
42 – LAUGH	92
43 – PHYSICAL ACTIVITY	94
44 – COMFORT ZONE	96
45 – RESPECT YOURSELF	98
46 – EDUCATE YOURSELF	100
47 – DELAYED GRATIFICATION	102
48 – AVOID NEGATIVE PEOPLE	104

49 – TIME MANAGEMENT 106
50 – ANGER MANAGEMENT 108
CONCLUSION 110
ABOUT THE AUTHOR..112

ACKNOWLEDGMENTS

I want to thank God (for answering my prayers when most needed), my wife, Dr. Saleema, (for being a pillar of strength in times of weakness), my sons Zeeshan & Faizan (for being the 'why' in my life), my parents Nasir & Dr. Safia (for teaching me resilience) and last but not least, my readers for taking the time to not only read my material but also for providing valuable feedback, inspiration, and motivation which encourages me to become a better writer and to provide high-quality content. Thank you!

1 - EXERCISE

Regular exercise can help reduce the symptoms of anxiety and depression in addition to medicine and therapy, which are both successful therapies for these diseases. Regular exercise may help reduce the symptoms of anxiety and depression in the following ways.

Benefits of Regular Exercise

Neurotransmitters: Exercise boosts the release of endorphins, serotonin, and dopamine, which are neurotransmitters that regulate mood and lessen anxiety and depressive symptoms. While serotonin and dopamine are linked to emotions of happiness and well-being, endorphins are natural painkillers that induce ecstasy.

Stress reduction: Exercise is a natural stress reducer. Exercise helps your body release tension and lower stress levels, which can help prevent sadness and anxiety. The stress hormone cortisol, which is frequently high in patients with anxiety and depression, can also be reduced by exercise.

Enhances sleep: Exercise can assist you to control your sleep cycles and raise the caliber of your slumber. Lack of sleep can worsen the signs of anxiety and sadness. Enough sleep is crucial for mental wellness.

Confidence: Exercise regularly can make you feel better about yourself, have more confidence, and have a better self-image. For those with depression, who frequently suffer with low self-esteem and self-worth, this can be extremely helpful.

Gives you a sense of direction: Including exercise in your daily routine can give you a sense of structure and direction, which is particularly beneficial for persons with depression who may have trouble motivating themselves and feeling lost.

Benefits of walking

Researchers have shown that walking can effectively reduce the signs of anxiety and depression. It is an easy technique to promote mental health because it is a low-impact activity that can be performed practically anyplace. Exercise causes our bodies to release endorphins, which are organic substances that help to lessen pain and improve happiness. Cortisol, a stress hormone that can worsen sadness and anxiety, can be reduced by walking. Walking outside also exposes you to nature and sunlight, both of which have been linked to improved mental health. Also, it can give a sense of achievement and serves as a diversion from unpleasant emotions and ideas. Overall, walking is a straightforward but effective method for enhancing mental health and general wellbeing.

Benefits of Strength Training

Strength training has been shown to improve mental health, particularly in easing the signs of anxiety and depression. Strength training, like walking, results in the production of endorphins, which can improve mood and lessen pain. Moreover, it can aid in lowering cortisol levels, which are linked to depression and anxiety. Strength training can also aid people in gaining a sense of control and self-efficacy, which boosts one's self-esteem and confidence. Also, it can enhance general cognitive performance and act as a beneficial diversion from unfavorable thoughts and emotions. Strength training can also enhance sleep quality, which has a positive effect on mental health. People can benefit from strength training on both a physical and mental health level by including it in a regular workout program.

Regular exercise is a highly effective method for reducing anxiety and depressive symptoms. Even a quick stroll or yoga practice can help lift your spirits and lower your stress levels - it doesn't have to be strenuous or time-consuming. Consider including regular exercise in your self-care routine if you experience anxiety or depression.

2 –SPEND TIME OUTDOORS

The simple yet powerful remedy for anxiety and depression is to spend time outside. A tranquil and serene setting like that found in nature can help to lower stress levels, elevate mood, and promote mental health. Here are a few ways why being outside might be good for your mental health.

First, being outside enables people to disconnect from the stress of daily life and commune with nature. According to studies, spending time outside helps reduce cortisol levels, a stress hormone linked to anxiety and depression. The release of feel-good hormones like dopamine and serotonin is also stimulated by being in nature, which can elevate mood and lessen depressive symptoms.

Second, physical activity, which has been demonstrated to have considerable positive effects on mental health, can include time spent outside. Endorphins, which are organic painkillers and mood enhancers, are produced more quickly when you exercise. Exercise has also been demonstrated to lessen the signs of depression and anxiety and enhance general mental health.

Lastly, being outside can give people a sense of accomplishment and purpose, which is particularly beneficial for those who are depressed. Hobbies like camping, gardening, and hiking can boost confidence and give people a sense of accomplishment.

Being outside has several advantages for one's mental health. Nature has a profound impact on our welfare, doing anything from lowering stress and anxiety to enhancing mood and encouraging physical exercise. Spending time in nature can therefore be an easy and effective method to enhance mental health and wellness, whether it be a trip through the woods or a leisurely stroll around the park.

3 - MINDFULNESS

It has been demonstrated that mindfulness, which is the discipline of being completely present and involved in the present moment without passing judgment, is an effective strategy for reducing anxiety and depression. People can free themselves from unhelpful thought patterns that fuel anxiety and sadness by concentrating on the here and now and monitoring their thoughts and feelings without getting sucked into them.

By fostering greater awareness and acceptance of one's thoughts and feelings, mindfulness can help those with anxiety and depression. Individuals might start to identify patterns that contribute to anxiety and depression when they are able to monitor their thoughts and feelings without passing judgment. By recognizing these patterns, people can create better coping mechanisms, such as cultivating self-compassion or employing cognitive-behavioral methods.

Moreover, mindfulness can aid people in gaining more resiliency and coping mechanisms. People can learn to accept painful thoughts and feelings without becoming overwhelmed by them by being completely present and involved in the moment. As a result, they will be able to better regulate their emotions, which will help them manage their anxiety and depression.

Also, mindfulness can support people in developing a stronger sense of self-awareness and self-compassion. People can learn to understand their own strengths and faults without self-criticism by being present and non-judgmental. This can lessen their emotions of worry and depression and help them form a more positive self-image.

Mindfulness can be a very effective approach for overcoming anxiety and sadness. People can learn to better manage their anxiety and depression and enhance their general well-being by improving their understanding and acceptance of their thoughts and feelings, strengthening their coping mechanisms and resilience, and raising their self-awareness and self-compassion.

4 - COGNITIVE BEHAVIORAL THERAPY

CBT is a form of psychotherapy that has been proven to be successful in treating a variety of mental health conditions, including anxiety and depression. The foundation of cognitive behavioral therapy (CBT) is the idea that our thoughts, feelings, and behaviors are interconnected and that altering our beliefs and behaviors can help lessen emotional suffering.

In cognitive behavioral therapy (CBT) for anxiety, the therapist works with the patient to identify and address harmful and unreasonable thoughts that fuel anxious sensations. Deep breathing exercises, progressive muscle relaxation, and exposure therapy—in which the patient is gradually exposed to the events or items that make them anxious—are some of the coping mechanisms that therapists use to help patients control anxiety symptoms. The patient is also taught how to identify and alter their unhelpful thought patterns, such as catastrophic thinking and black-and-white thinking, which can increase anxiety symptoms, as part of CBT.

Therapists also assist their patients with CBT for depression by helping them recognize and challenge negative and self-defeating ideas that contribute to feelings of hopelessness and despair. The therapist aids the patient in learning strategies for enhancing good experiences, such as planning fun activities, and recognizing and altering negative thought patterns that lead to depressive symptoms, such as self-blame and critical self-talk.

CBT has been proven to be a successful treatment for depression and anxiety, and some studies even suggest that it is just as beneficial as using medication to treat these illnesses. Most patients see a significant reduction in their symptoms within 12 to 20 sessions of CBT, making it another treatment option that is quite brief in duration.

CBT provides a methodical, scientifically supported method of treating anxiety and depression that encourages patients to actively participate in their own recovery. CBT can help patients reduce emotional discomfort and enhance their overall quality of life by educating them on how to alter their thoughts and behaviors.

5 – JOIN A SUPPORT GROUP

Becoming involved in a support group can be a very effective way to deal with anxiety and depression which are frequently isolating illnesses that can make people feel helpless and alone. People can connect with others who can relate to what they're going through, share their stories, and get emotional support in a support group.

Joining a support group may help lessen feelings of loneliness and isolation, which is one of the main advantages. Many people who struggle with anxiety and depression may believe they are the only ones, but a support group can give them a sense of connection and belonging. People might receive validation for their feelings and lessen feelings of guilt and stigma by getting in touch with people who have had similar experiences.

Moreover, support groups can offer useful coping mechanisms for handling anxiety and depression. Members can share methods that have helped them, such as mindfulness meditation, physical activity, or self-care routines. These methods can give people a sense of empowerment and control over their mental health.

Support groups can also aid in enhancing one's sense of value and self-esteem. People can feel more secure in their ability to manage their mental health when they get support and encouragement from others. Support groups can also give members the chance to lend a hand to others, which can heighten feelings of fulfillment and purpose.

Folks who are battling anxiety and depression may find great benefit from attending a support group. Individuals can connect with others who understand what they're going through and share their stories in a secure and encouraging environment. Consider finding a local support group or an online community to assist you on your road to recovery if you're dealing with anxiety or depression.

6 - JOURNAL

It is well known fact that journaling is a crucial therapeutic practice which may help people manage their anxiety and depression. People can better understand their emotions, manage stress, and enhance their general mental health by putting their ideas, feelings, and experiences in writing.

By giving people a secure and private place to express themselves, journaling helps reduce anxiety and sadness, among other symptoms. Those who find it difficult to share their negative feelings and thoughts with others might release them through writing. The cathartic nature of this method may aid in easing any anxiety or depression that people may be going through.

Also, keeping a journal might help people spot trends and triggers that lead to their anxiety and sadness. People might start to identify recurring themes or circumstances that might be causing them to encounter mental health difficulties by writing down their thoughts and experiences. This knowledge can be empowering and encourage people to take action to manage their symptoms by addressing these triggers.

Journaling can assist people in reframing unfavorable thoughts and feelings into more uplifting and productive viewpoints. People can question and reframe their negative views into more constructive ones by putting them on paper. This cognitive restructuring may lessen the intensity and occurrence of negative thoughts while also enhancing general mental health.

Keeping a journal can help you manage your anxiety and depression. Journaling can enhance general mental health and well-being by giving people a secure and private place for self-expression, assisting them in recognizing patterns and triggers, and enabling the cognitive rewiring of negative thoughts.

7 – PAINTING, DRAWING, COLORING

In the human psyche, art has long been known to have positive therapeutic effects that include lowering anxiety and sadness. Art activities like painting, drawing, and coloring can all provide people a way to express themselves, unwind, and feel in control, which helps lessen the symptoms of anxiety and depression.

When making art, the act of concentrating on a task and expressing oneself via color, form, and composition may be contemplative and peaceful, assisting in promoting relaxation and lowering anxiety. While allowing an artist to produce something real and significant, this process also gives the artist a sense of control, which can increase confidence and self-esteem.

Practicing art might cause the release of endorphins, which are neurotransmitters that can lessen stress and elevate happiness. The symptoms of depression, which are frequently characterized by a lack of drive, enjoyment, and energy, may be lessened by doing this.

Mindfulness meditation, which has been demonstrated to be useful in lowering anxiety and depression, can be practiced through drawing, painting, and coloring. People can become more aware of their thoughts and emotions by concentrating on the here and now and the task at hand, which can help to lessen feelings of being overwhelmed and encourage a sense of calmness.

It has been demonstrated that art therapy, which is working with a qualified therapist to make art as a way of exploring emotions and fostering healing, is successful in lowering anxiety and depression. Individuals can express themselves in a secure and encouraging setting with this method, and they can also gain understanding of their feelings and thoughts.

Creative activities like painting, drawing, and coloring may be quite effective in lowering anxiety and depression, giving one a sense of control, encouraging relaxation and awareness, and inducing endorphin release. These advantages make art, whether it is performed alone or in conjunction with therapy, a vital supplement to any mental health treatment strategy.

8 - MUSIC

It's well known that music has a profound emotional regulatory effect and may help those with anxiety and depression. Research has shown that music therapy can be useful in easing symptoms and elevating mood and is frequently used as an adjunctive treatment for anxiety and depression.

Music can help alleviate anxiety and depression. Dopamine, a neurotransmitter linked to pleasure and reward, is released when we listen to music we appreciate. Dopamine can help us manage our emotions and lessen anxiety and depressive symptoms.

Music not only alters brain chemistry but also acts as a deterrent from unfavorable feelings and thoughts. As we listen to music, our attention is diverted from our anxieties and concerns and instead is drawn to the sounds and rhythms. This can aid in ending the loop of self-talk and ruminating that frequently accompanies anxiety and depression.

Moreover, music can foster a sense of community and connection. We frequently feel a sense of shared experience with others who like the same songs or genres when we listen to music. This sense of connection may help those who experience loneliness or isolation.

Music can be a means of expression and emotional release. Many people discover that making or listening to music enables them to communicate emotions that they might not be able to verbalize. This may be a potent method for processing and overcoming challenging emotions.

Listening to music can help those with anxiety and depression. Music has the capacity to uplift our mood and enhance our emotional wellbeing.

9 – FUN ACTIVITIES

While there are many therapies available, including therapy and medication, engaging in enjoyable activities can also help to reduce the symptoms of anxiety and depression.

Fun activities can make people feel more at ease and content, which can lessen the stress, worry, and sadness that come with anxiety and depression. The body's inherent feel-good chemicals called endorphins are released when participating in enjoyable activities. This may result in a happier disposition and a stronger sense of wellbeing.

Entertaining activities can also be used to divert attention from unfavorable feelings and ideas. People are less prone to concentrate on negative thoughts, which can increase the symptoms of anxiety and depression, when they are engaged in an enjoyable activity. Participating in activities with others can also foster a sense of community and social support, both of which can enhance mental health.

A person may love several kinds of activities. It might be anything, from physical activity and sports to artistic endeavors like writing, performing music, or painting. Others like indoor pursuits like reading or playing video games, while some people find that outdoor pursuits like hiking or gardening help them feel peaceful and relaxed.

Engaging in enjoyable activities may help to reduce the signs and symptoms of anxiety and depression. The effects of participating in enjoyable activities include mood improvement, distraction from unfavorable thoughts, social support, and a sense of community. As a result, people who are struggling with anxiety or depression are urged to choose activities that make them happy and to engage in them.

10 – CONNECT WITH A PERSON YOU TRUST

Having a relationship with a reliable individual can help you manage your anxiety and depression. It might be challenging to deal with strong emotions of concern or despair on our own but we can experience a sense of comfort and support when we reach out to someone we trust.

We may express our emotions in a secure, nonjudgmental setting when we connect with a trustworthy individual, which is one of the reasons why trustworthy individuals may assist with anxiety and depression. We feel heard and acknowledged when we express our thoughts and feelings to someone we trust. This can help us gain perspective and lessen the intensity of our feelings.

Speaking with a reliable source can also provide a fresh perspective on our predicament. A dependable friend or relative may be able to provide a new viewpoint or propose coping mechanisms that we might not have thought of on our own. This can make us feel like we have greater control over our emotions and are better able to handle them in the future.

Feelings of loneliness and isolation, which are frequent for people with anxiety and depression, might be lessened by connecting with a dependable person. We are more inclined to feel optimistic about the future and less overburdened by our present circumstances when we see that we are not alone in our problems.

Talking to a reliable person can help you manage your anxiety and depression. We can make efforts to feel more in charge of our mental health by expressing our feelings in a safe and encouraging atmosphere, learning new information, and experiencing less loneliness. If you require assistance with anxiety or depression, think about talking to a dependable friend, member of your family, or mental health expert.

11 – SEEK COUNSELING

Counseling, usually referred to as talk therapy, is a type of therapy that can aid those who are experiencing anxiety and depression. It entails having discussions and exploring emotions, thoughts, and behaviors with a qualified mental health practitioner, like a counselor or therapist. Several studies have shown that counseling can help people with anxiety and depression.

By offering a secure and accepting environment in which to communicate one's feelings and emotions, counseling can help those with anxiety and depression. This can be especially beneficial for people who do not have a support structure or do not feel comfortable opening up to loved ones about their emotions. The therapist can provide affirmation and empathy, which can lessen feelings of isolation and loneliness.

Therapy can also assist people in recognizing harmful thought patterns and actions that can be causing their anxiety or depression. The therapist can offer techniques and resources to assist the patient in confronting and changing these negative thoughts with more constructive ones. A greater sense of control over one's emotions and thoughts might result from this, which helps lessen feelings of helplessness and hopelessness.

Counseling can also assist people in learning coping mechanisms for dealing with anxiety and depressive symptoms. These can include problem-solving approaches, relaxation exercises, and mindfulness practices. People might feel more in control of their mental health and more confident in their capacity to deal with difficult situations by learning how to regulate their symptoms.

Keep in mind that all therapists and counselors are not the same. So if you feel you're not able to connect with your therapist, move on to another one until you find a good fit. Fighting anxiety and depression is an active process and requires time, patience and commitment. Stick with your treatment and there will come a point in your progress where you will look back and say to yourself, "I'm never going back there again!" ☐

Counseling can be a very successful method of treating anxiety and depression. People can explore their emotions and learn coping mechanisms in a secure, encouraging setting, which promotes a stronger sense of control and wellbeing.

12 – DEEP BREATHING EXERCISES

Exercises that involve deep breathing can be an effective strategy for reducing anxiety and depressive symptoms. These methods support the body's autonomic nervous system, which regulates automatic processes including respiration, digestion, and heart rate. We activate the parasympathetic nervous system when we breathe deeply and deliberately, which blocks the fight-or-flight response brought on by stress and anxiety.

The fact that deep breathing exercises slow down the breath and encourage relaxation is one of its main advantages. Our tendency to breathe quickly and shallowly when we're anxious or depressed can make these symptoms worse. We may lessen the body's response to stress, lower our heart rate and blood pressure, and feel more at ease by taking long, deep breaths.

Deep breathing exercises also have the potential to enhance concentration and mental clarity. It's simple for our minds to wander and lose focus when we're feeling anxious or depressed. Deep breathing exercises help us focus on the present moment rather than our rushing thoughts, which can make us feel more centered and grounded.

Deep breathing exercises have also been found in research to help with mood enhancement and depression symptom reduction. By increasing oxygen flow to the brain, deep breathing can help increase levels of neurotransmitters like serotonin and dopamine, which are linked to positive emotions like happiness and wellbeing.

Deep breathing exercises are a quick and efficient technique to reduce anxiety and depressive symptoms. These practices can add value to any self-care regimen by slowing the breath, encouraging relaxation, enhancing mental clarity, and elevating our mood.

13 – SET GOALS

The ability to set objectives can be a very effective strategy for overcoming anxiety and depression. Those who struggle with these conditions frequently feel powerless over their lives, which can produce feelings of helplessness and hopelessness. Individuals can take charge of their life and find a feeling of direction and purpose by creating clear, attainable goals. As a result, anxiety and depression may be lessened.

Individuals gain a sense of direction and purpose from their goals. Setting goals fundamentally involves making a road plan for oneself thereby creating an awareness not only of goals but steps required to achieve those goals. Particularly for someone who feels lost or caught in a rut, this may be immensely powerful. People are more inclined to act and strive towards a goal if they have a clear aim in sight as opposed to feeling helpless and paralyzed by their own worry or sadness.

Goals also provide people with a feeling of satisfaction and success. When you set a goal and accomplish it, you feel proud and satisfied. This is crucial for those who are depressed because it can be challenging to find enjoyment or pleasure in routine activities. The good feeling surge that comes from achieving a goal might assist to balance out the negative emotions linked to anxiety and depression.

Goal setting is a potent technique for reducing anxiety and depression. Goals can help people take charge of their life and find a road ahead toward a happier, more satisfying future by giving them a sense of purpose, direction, and accomplishment.

14 – SLEEP WELL

Maintaining excellent mental health requires getting a good night's sleep. Sleeping gives our brains a chance to rest and repair, which can have a big impact on how we feel emotionally. Poor sleep may worsen anxiety and depression. There are several advantages to getting enough sleep that can help relieve symptoms.

First off, sleep is essential for controlling our mood. Our brains are more likely to overreact to unfavorable stimuli when we are sleep deprived, which increases our feelings of anxiety and depression. On the other hand, when we get adequate sleep, our brains are better equipped to process emotions and manage our reactions to stress, which lowers our risk of experiencing depressive and anxious feelings.

Sleep is essential for preserving our physical well-being, which in turn can enhance our mental well-being. Lack of sleep causes our bodies to create more cortisol and other stress hormones, which can raise anxiety and sadness. Contrarily, getting adequate sleep helps support the regulation of these hormones and support a more balanced, healthy body.

Sleep is crucial for cognitive processes including decision-making and memory. We are more equipped to deal with life's problems, especially those that can fuel emotions of anxiety and despair, when we are well-rested.

A restful night's sleep is essential for preserving excellent mental health. Our emotional health may benefit from its ability to better manage our mood, support physical health, and enhance cognitive ability. Making sleep a priority and creating healthy sleeping habits are worthwhile if you experience anxiety or depression since they can help you control your symptoms.

15 – YOGA

Since it has been around for thousands of years, yoga is an age-old activity that is well-known for its advantages in lowering stress. Two of the most prevalent mental health issues are anxiety and depression, both of which can significantly lower a person's quality of life. Yoga can be a useful tool for easing the signs of anxiety and depression.

Yoga's emphasis on relaxation is one strategy for easing anxiety and depression. Yoga consists of a set of postures, breathing exercises, and meditation that help the body and mind to calm down and unwind. Our bodies can stiffen up and our minds can race with unpleasant ideas when we're anxious or depressed. The practice of yoga aids in easing muscular tension, and its emphasis on breathing helps to relax the mind and calm the body.

Yoga not only encourages relaxation but also lifts one's spirits. According to studies, yoga can boost the brain's synthesis of feel-good neurotransmitters like serotonin and dopamine. The increased synthesis of these chemicals, which are linked to feelings of joy and wellbeing, can aid in reducing the signs and symptoms of anxiety and depression.

Yoga also alleviates anxiety and depression by encouraging mindfulness. The practice of mindfulness involves being in the present and objectively monitoring one's thoughts and feelings. Negative emotions and thoughts can feed anxiety and depression, and practicing mindfulness can help to stop the cycle of negative thinking. In order to quiet the mind and lessen the influence of negative ideas, yoga promotes mindfulness by encouraging attention to the present moment and breathing.

Practicing yoga is quite effective for lowering anxiety and depression. Yoga offers a comprehensive approach to mental health that can be advantageous for people of all ages and fitness levels by fostering relaxation, elevating mood, and increasing mindfulness.

16 – VOLUNTEER

A great method to enhance mental health and wellbeing is through volunteering. At some point in their life, many people deal with anxiety and sadness, and volunteering can be a helpful outlet for these emotions. Volunteering can provide people with a sense of purpose and perspective by helping them focus on the needs of others, which helps lessen the symptoms of anxiety and depression.

By fostering a sense of social connectivity, volunteering can help with anxiety and sadness. Those who struggle with anxiety and depression frequently feel alone and cut off from others. Volunteering enables people to socialize and form connections with others, which can lessen feelings of isolation and loneliness. Also, volunteering can foster a sense of community and belonging that can lessen the effects of sadness.

Volunteering can boost a person's self-esteem and sense of success. Many individuals who deal with anxiety and depression contend with thoughts of inadequate self-worth. People can feel a sense of purpose and accomplishment by volunteering and giving back to their community, and this can boost their confidence and self-esteem.

Volunteering can offer a feeling of routine and structure, which is beneficial for people who battle anxiety and depression. Giving back to the community can bring stability and regularity, which helps lessen feelings of anxiety and being overwhelmed.

As a strong remedy for feelings of hopelessness and despair, volunteering can also give people a sense of meaning and purpose. People can find a sense of purpose and direction in their life by helping others and giving back to their community, which can lessen the symptoms of depression.

Overall, those who struggle with anxiety and depression may find it helpful to volunteer. Volunteering can assist people's mental health and well-being by fostering social connections, a sense of achievement and self-worth, structure and regularity, and a sense of meaning and purpose.

17 – AROMATHERAPY

Aromatherapy is a holistic treatment method that uses plant-based essential oils to support mental, emotional, and spiritual health. It is a well-liked alternative therapy used to treat a variety of health issues, including anxiety and depression.

The therapeutic advantages of aromatherapy are founded on the idea that essential oils contain a plant's life force, which has the power to influence the energy system of the body and encourage recovery. Essential oils interact with the limbic system of the brain, which regulates emotions, memory, and behavior, when breathed or applied topically.

Many studies have demonstrated the potent relief of anxiety and depressive symptoms by specific essential oils. The most widely used essential oils for this are lavender, chamomile, bergamot, and ylang-ylang.

It's commonly known that lavender oil has calming and relaxing qualities. According to studies, inhaling lavender oil might lower anxiety and enhance sleep. Because it has a calming and relaxing impact on the body, chamomile oil is also good at relieving the symptoms of anxiety.

Another essential oil that can help with depressive symptoms is bergamot oil. Its cheerful and zesty aroma can improve mood and lessen stress. Ylang-ylang oil has a relaxing impact on the nervous system and can encourage feelings of joy and happiness, making it useful for treating the symptoms of depression.

Aromatherapy is a secure and organic technique to reduce the signs of anxiety and depression. Modern research has validated the therapeutic benefits of essential oils, which have been utilized for centuries. Consider adding aromatherapy as a supplemental therapy to your current treatment plan if you struggle with anxiety or depression. Before using essential oils, always seek the advice of a licensed aromatherapist or healthcare professional, especially if you have any underlying medical concerns or are pregnant.

18 – STAY AWAY FROM DRUGS

Anxiety and depression are only two of the many mental health conditions that drug misuse is frequently associated with. There is a widely held view that while drug usage may temporarily numb unpleasant emotions, over time it may exacerbate mental health issues. Thus, abstaining from narcotics can lessen the feelings of anxiety and depression.

Many factors, including genetic predisposition, environmental conditions, and previous experiences, can contribute to anxiety and depression. By changing the chemical equilibrium of the brain, drugs can temporarily numb these unpleasant feelings and may result in long-term modifications to brain chemistry and psychological well-being.

According to research, substance addiction can alter the brain's reward circuit, which can result in enduring emotions of worry and sadness. The ability of the brain to control emotions can be damaged by drugs like marijuana and opioids, which increases the risk of mental health disorders. Drug misuse can also worsen social isolation and a lack of motivation.

On the other hand, folks who are depressed or anxious can reap many advantages from refraining from drug use. People can avoid the temporary relief that drugs offer by abstaining from them and instead learn more effective coping skills. Therapy, physical activity, and mindfulness exercises are a few examples of things that can help with mental health.

Drug usage can exacerbate the symptoms of anxiety and depression, but abstaining from drugs can alleviate these symptoms. Long-term improvements in mental health and general well-being can result from learning healthy coping skills and getting expert assistance.

19 – BALANCED DIET & STAY HYDRATED

Balanced Diet

A balanced diet is essential for preserving excellent physical health, but it also significantly affects mental wellness. According to research, our diets can significantly influence how much anxiety and depressive symptoms we experience. Here are a few ways that a balanced diet might lessen anxiety and depression.

A balanced diet that includes whole foods like fruits, vegetables, lean proteins, and whole grains gives our bodies the critical elements they require to function effectively. B vitamins, magnesium, zinc, and omega-3 fatty acids are some of these nutrients, and research has shown that they can lessen the signs and symptoms of anxiety and depression.

The following are some benefits of following a balanced diet.

Controls blood sugar levels: Unstable blood sugar levels can cause irritation, anxiety, and mood changes. A balanced diet rich in protein, fiber, and complex carbs can help control blood sugar levels and minimize the spikes and crashes that can lead to anxiety and depression.

Reduces inflammation: An increased incidence of depression and anxiety has been related to inflammation in the body. An anti-inflammatory diet that contains foods like fruits, vegetables, nuts, and fatty fish can help the body fight inflammation and elevate mood.

Improves intestinal health: A healthy stomach can contribute to better mental health, according to studies on the gut-brain connection, a field of research that is expanding. Eating a balanced diet that includes fermented foods like yogurt, kimchi, and sauerkraut, will not only lessen the symptoms of anxiety and depression but will also result in a healthy gut flora.

Maintaining a healthy diet is crucial for easing the signs of anxiety and depression. A balanced diet can support healthy mental health and general well-being by supplying necessary nutrients, controlling blood sugar levels, lowering inflammation, and enhancing gastrointestinal health.

Stay Hydrated

In addition to being critical for your mental health, staying hydrated is also crucial for sustaining good physical health. Dehydration can cause several symptoms, including fatigue, headaches, and irritability, that can aggravate anxiety and depression. Being hydrated can help with anxiety and depression in the following ways.

Improves mood: Feelings of weariness and lethargy brought on by dehydration can lead to sadness. Water consumption can increase energy levels, elevate mood, and lessen depression symptoms.

Reduces anxiety: Heart palpitations, vertigo, and shortness of breath are just a few of the symptoms of anxiety that can be brought on by dehydration. Being hydrated can aid in easing these sensations and lowering anxiety levels.

Enhances cognitive function: Dehydration can affect one's ability to remember things, pay attention to things, and make decisions. These processes can be enhanced by staying hydrated, which makes it easier to control stress and lessen anxiety and depressive symptoms.

Flushes out toxins: Water consumption aids in the removal of toxins from the body, particularly those that may be responsible for depression and anxiety. Staying hydrated prevents these toxins from accumulating and in turn decreases signs of anxiety and depression.

Regulates hormones: Hormones that control stress and mood might be affected by dehydration. In order to keep hormones in balance and lessen the signs of anxiety and depression, it is important to stay hydrated.

Maintaining excellent mental health requires being hydrated. You can decrease the signs of anxiety and depression, elevate your mood, enhance your cognitive abilities, and control your hormone levels by drinking adequate water. Hence, make sure you're getting enough water each day to promote your mental wellbeing.

20 – TOXIC PEOPLE & TOXIC FAMILY

Toxic People

Those that are toxic affect others negatively and create dysfunction in their surroundings. They frequently engage in emotional sapping, manipulation, and control. It's crucial to detect the warning signals of toxic conduct in others and learn how to protect yourself since spending time with toxic people may be detrimental to your mental and emotional well-being.

People that are toxic frequently exhibit a lack of empathy for others and are self-centered. To exert control over those around them, they could employ emotional manipulation techniques like guilt-tripping or gaslighting. Moreover, toxic people may be highly judgmental and critical of others and may work to lower others' self-esteem.

Another characteristic shared by toxic individuals is an excessive need for control and demand. If their wishes are not fulfilled, they may get irritated or aggressive and attempt to control how others should act, think, or feel. Also, they could be quick to judge and condemn others and use derogatory words to establish their superiority.

Being in a relationship with a toxic person can be particularly harmful since they may try to keep their partner away from friends and family or resort to emotional abuse to keep control. It's crucial to get assistance and support from dependable friends, family members, or mental health experts if you believe you are in a toxic relationship.

Set healthy boundaries and engage in self-care in order to safeguard yourself against toxic people. This may entail cutting back on interactions with toxic people, developing the ability to refuse requests when required, and putting more of an emphasis on relationships and activities that are uplifting and joyful. In the end, it is up to each person to decide the types of relationships and interactions they are prepared to put up with and to take precautions to safeguard their own mental and emotional health.

Toxic Family

Family members can harm you in several ways, including psychologically, emotionally, and even violently. In certain cases, the same people who are supposed to be your support system actually contribute to your suffering.

One of the most frequent ways that family members can harm you is emotionally. This can involve actions like manipulation, neglect, or verbal abuse. Insults, put-downs, and even screaming matches can all be considered forms of verbal abuse. Neglect can take the shape of disregarding your needs, failing to show you love or attention, or even failing to be there for you when you need someone. Although manipulation can take many different forms, it typically entails someone attempting to exert undue control or influence over you.

Another way that family can harm you is psychologically. This may involve techniques like gaslighting, in which a person tries to undermine your sense of reality, or it might even involve denying that you have mental health issues or telling you that you're crazy. Continual criticism, defamation, or even unfavorable comparisons to others might also fall under this category.

Finally, family members may harm you physically. Physical abuse, negligence, or even just failing to take good care of you are examples of this. From beating or punching to more serious acts of violence, physical abuse can take many different forms. Neglect can take the form of failing to give you the right nutrition or medical attention or failing to keep you safe from harm.

It's crucial to keep in mind that not all families are like this and that there are constructive methods to handle this kind of circumstance. You can safeguard yourself from the harm that family can bring about by seeking professional assistance, establishing boundaries, or even severing ties with toxic relatives.

How to deal with Toxic Family Members

It might be challenging and complicated to deal with toxic family members, but it's crucial to put your own physical and mental health first. Here are some guidelines for dealing with negative relatives.

Establishing boundaries is one of the most crucial measures in coping with toxic family members. This entails setting up clear guidelines for the behavior you will and will not put up with from them. Tell them what actions are prohibited and what will happen if they do so again. Be firm but courteous while maintaining your boundaries.

Seek support. When coping with toxic family members, it's critical to have a support system. This can be a support group, a therapist, or pals. It can make you feel less alone and more in control to be surrounded by people who acknowledge and understand your emotions.

Self-care is important. Make sure you give your personal well-being and care top priority. This can involve engaging in regular exercise, eating a nutritious diet, and obtaining enough sleep. Take part in things that make you happy, relax you, and give you a sense of satisfaction.

Examine treatment. Dealing with toxic family members might be facilitated by therapy. A therapist can offer direction and support as you negotiate challenging family dynamics and assist you in creating coping mechanisms to control stress and anxiety.

Cut connections or limit contact. In some circumstances, it could be important to cut ties or restrict contact with toxic family members. It can be challenging to choose, but it's crucial to put your own physical and mental health first. Before making this choice, think about chatting with a trustworthy friend or therapist.

Although coping with toxic family members might be difficult, it's crucial to put your own physical and mental health first. Get help, establish boundaries, take care of yourself, think about counseling, and make the choices that are right for you.

21 – CUT CAFFEINE

Coffee, tea, and soft drinks all contain caffeine, a common stimulant. Caffeine is well known for improving mental clarity and focus, yet it can also be harmful to mental health. According to studies, caffeine can make some people feel anxious or depressed, especially those who habitually drink excessive amounts of the substance.

Caffeine withdrawal can help with the symptoms of anxiety and depression. This is because caffeine stimulates the central nervous system, which can elevate blood pressure, heart rate, and the release of stress hormones like cortisol. Overdosing on coffee can make it difficult to fall asleep and lead to agitation, mood fluctuations, and uneasiness.

According to research, people who consume less coffee had fewer symptoms of anxiety and depression. According to a study in the Journal of Psychiatric Research, people who drink a lot of coffee have a higher chance of acquiring anxiety problems. Another study indicated that cutting back on caffeine can significantly boost mood and lower anxiety levels. This study was also published in the Journal of Affective Disorders.

Moreover, coffee may reduce the effectiveness of several drugs used to treat anxiety and depression. Some antidepressants may be less successful at treating the symptoms of depression because caffeine can reduce their absorption.

While caffeine might temporarily enhance energy levels, consuming too much of it can have detrimental effects on mental health. Limiting caffeine intake can assist in relieving these symptoms and enhance general mental health. It's crucial to keep in mind that everyone reacts to caffeine differently, so it may be necessary to try out various doses to discover the optimal one for you.

22 – LIMIT ALCOHOL

The symptoms of anxiety and depression can be significantly reduced by limiting alcohol consumption. Alcohol depresses the central nervous system and has several negative effects on mental health, including anxiety and depression.

Alcohol can temporarily calm the body when ingested in moderation, resulting in a relaxed sensation and lessened inhibitions. The body's capacity to control moods and emotions can be compromised by excessive alcohol use, which can exacerbate feelings of anxiety and depression.

According to studies, excessive alcohol users are more likely to struggle with depression and anxiety symptoms. This is because alcohol can change the ratio of neurotransmitters in the brain, including dopamine and serotonin, which are crucial for controlling mood.

Alcohol can also alter sleep patterns, which can result in feelings of exhaustion, irritability, and depression and may prevent the body from absorbing vital nutrients like magnesium and vitamin B12, which are essential for preserving mental health.

By minimizing their likelihood of experiencing anxiety and depression, people can enhance their mental health by limiting their alcohol consumption which may result in more restful sleep, more vitality, and enhanced mood.

Those who experience anxiety or depression may discover that restricting their alcohol consumption might help them better control their symptoms. They can look into other methods, such as exercise, mindfulness, or therapy, to enhance their mental health rather than using alcohol as a coping technique.

Restricting alcohol consumption can significantly improve mental health by lowering the likelihood of experiencing anxiety and depression, enhancing sleep, and boosting energy. Prioritize your mental health and, if necessary, get help from a professional.

23 – LIMIT TIME ON SOCIAL MEDIA

Modern life has evolved at an alarming rate and is significantly impacted by social media, which gives us rapid access to news, information, and the most recent updates from our friends and family. Social media does offer some advantages, but it can also be bad for our mental health. According to research, excessive social media use is linked to sadness, anxiety, and a decline in happiness and life satisfaction.

Limiting the amount of time we spend on social media is one practical way to lessen the detrimental effects it has on our mental health. We can lessen our exposure to potentially hazardous content and damaging social comparisons by establishing clear time limits for social media use. By allowing us to concentrate on other elements of our lives that are more rewarding and important, this can help us feel less anxious and depressed.

The "fear of missing out" (FOMO) that is frequently linked to constant social media use can also be avoided by restricting our use of social media. Our continual scanning of social media feeds might make us agitated and anxious about what we might be missing out on, which raises our anxiety and depressive symptoms. We can relieve ourselves of this ongoing strain and concentrate on the here and now by restricting how much time we spend on social media.

One simple exercise is to lay your phone upside down on the table so that the screen is facing the table. Set a timer for 5 minutes, and do not touch your phone. As you get better, gradually increase the time. This exercise will help you control your urges to keep checking your phone. Like everything in life, practice makes perfect.

Restricting our usage of social media can support our efforts to develop a sense of presence and mindfulness in our daily activities. We can improve our emotional control and sense of self-awareness by turning off social media and concentrating on our own experiences and relationships with others. By reducing the symptoms of anxiety and sadness, this can ultimately result in better emotions of happiness and wellbeing.

24 – PRACTICE SELF-CARE

Millions of people worldwide are afflicted by the two main mental health disorders of anxiety and depression. Neglecting self-care is one of the main causes of their growth, while there are other variables as well. Taking intentional steps to enhance your physical, mental, and emotional wellbeing is known as self-care. It can lessen the signs of anxiety and depression and perhaps stop them from starting when performed regularly.

Self-care can take many different forms, such as physical activity, a balanced diet, mindfulness, and enough sleep. By releasing endorphins during physical activity, for example, you can control anxiety and depression. Endorphins are organic mood enhancers. Exercise can also boost your confidence, give you a sense of accomplishment, and calm you—all of which are crucial for lowering anxiety and depression.

Another important aspect of self-care is maintaining a healthy, balanced diet. Nutrient-dense foods, such as fruits, vegetables, whole grains, and lean proteins, can offer the vitamins and minerals required to support brain health and mood regulation. On the other hand, eating processed meals, drinking sugary beverages, and drinking too much coffee can make anxiety and depression symptoms worse.

Deep breathing, yoga, and mindfulness exercises can all aid with anxiety and depression relief. These leisurely pursuits foster reflection, self-awareness, and relaxation, all of which can lessen the symptoms of anxiety and depression.

Getting enough sleep is an essential component of self-care that can help reduce the symptoms of anxiety and depression. Lack of sleep can worsen the signs of anxiety and depression because sleep is essential for mood regulation. A regular sleep schedule and excellent sleeping habits can encourage sound sleep and elevate mood.

Taking care of oneself can greatly lessen the symptoms of anxiety and depression. A person's total quality of life can be improved by putting their physical, mental, and emotional well-being first. This will help them feel less stressed and more resilient.

25 – TAKE A BATH

A quick and efficient technique to ease anxiety and depression is to take a bath. There are several ways that taking a bath can make you feel peaceful and relaxed, which helps lessen the signs of anxiety and depression.

First off, taking a warm bath can assist to reduce joint and muscular strain. This physical unwinding can aid in lowering stress and anxiety symptoms, which are frequently accompanied by tension in various parts of the body. Also, the warmth of the water may aid in boosting blood flow, which may help to induce relaxation.

Second, taking a bath can also help you feel relaxed mentally. A reprieve from the commotion of daily life can be found in the quiet and tranquil setting of a bath. For people who are dealing with anxiety or depression, this quiet time might allow for thought and introspection.

A bath's relaxing effects may be increased by adding aromatherapy. It has been demonstrated that some smells, like lavender, can relax the body and the mind. A bath can be made to have a calming and therapeutic effect by adding bath salts or essential oils.

Finally, you might find taking a bath to be nurturing to your overall health. Self-care practices can be a potent weapon in the fight against anxiety and depression and can support the development of a sense of wellbeing and self-worth.

Bathing might be a quick and easy technique to ease anxiety and depression. A bath can bring physical and mental relaxation, aromatherapy, and a sense of self-care, all of which can help one feel more at ease and relaxed.

26 – POSITIVE AFFIRMATIONS

Simple but effective words known as positive affirmations can ease anxiety and depression. They are a type of self-talk that emphasizes constructive ideas and convictions. People can alter their perspective and attitude by repeatedly saying these affirmations, which can result in better mental health.

Millions of people throughout the world suffer from the prevalent mental health conditions of anxiety and depression. They may be brought on by several things, including stress, trauma, and genetics. These situations can become worse as a result of negative ideas and attitudes, which can then fuel a vicious cycle of bad behavior. By encouraging positive thoughts and beliefs, positive affirmations can aid in breaking this pattern.

Positive affirmations are repeated over and over, which develops new neural connections in the brain. Positive thoughts and beliefs are reinforced by these pathways, which over time make them easier to access and automate. This can help overcome unfavorable ideas and assumptions that cause anxiety and depression. You may have seen tennis players talking to themselves after missing a shot. They are tapping into the power of positive affirmations which are known to boost confidence and self-esteem, both of which can enhance mental health.

Positive affirmations come in a variety of forms that people can implement to overcome anxiety and depression. The following are a few examples.

"I can handle everything that comes my way."

"I am deserving of respect and love."

"I choose to concentrate on the good aspects of my life."

"I am appreciative of what I have."

"I have control over my ideas and feelings."

These affirmations can be spoken out or silently repeated, and they can be altered to meet the requirements and circumstances of each person. They can be applied at any time, including when rising in the morning, right before bed, or in times of stress.

Using positive affirmations to relieve anxiety and depression is a quick and efficient method. People can enhance their mental health and general wellbeing by encouraging positive thoughts and attitudes.

27 – BE ORGANIZED

An effective approach for reducing anxiety and depressive symptoms is being organized. While an orderly workplace can provide a sense of serenity and control, a cluttered setting can lead to feelings of overload and stress. These are a few ways that being organized can lessen anxiety and depression.

Reduced Clutter: A clutter-free environment is less likely to be a source of tension and worry. A sense of turmoil and disorder brought on by cluttered areas can make people feel overwhelmed and out of control. You may make your space feel calmer and more serene by arranging and decluttering it.

Enhanced Efficiency: When you are organized, you use your time and energy more effectively. You are aware of where everything is and have quick access to it whenever you need it. You won't have to waste time looking for things or stressing over forgetting anything crucial, which can help lower stress and anxiety.

Better Time Management: Being organized might help you in scheduling and managing your time more effectively. This can make you feel like you have more control over your life and feel less anxious and overwhelmed. You may manage your time more effectively and feel less stressed by establishing goals and priorities, and then making a strategy to achieve them.

Improved Mental Health: Research has shown that depression and anxiety can be exacerbated by a cluttered atmosphere. You may cultivate a sense of order and control that can support good mental health by organizing your space. Furthermore, arranging can be therapeutic and aid in lowering stress and anxiety.

Being organized is a useful technique for reducing anxiety and depressive symptoms. Being organized can help you feel in control of your life by eliminating clutter, boosting efficiency, enhancing time management, and fostering good mental health.

28 – DAILY ROUTINE

Common mental health issues like anxiety and depression may influence a person's wellbeing and quality of life. While there are many ways to address anxiety and depression, creating a regular routine can help to reduce symptoms and enhance mental health.

Setting a regular schedule for tasks like waking up, exercising, eating, working, and sleeping is part of a daily routine. People can give their life structure and predictability by developing routines, which helps lessen feelings of worry and despair. The ability to regulate one's day through a routine can be powerful and lessen emotions of helplessness.

A daily schedule can also encourage good habits that have been proven to enhance mental health. Regular exercise, for instance, has been demonstrated to lessen the signs and symptoms of anxiety and depression by increasing endorphins and lowering stress chemicals in the body. People can enhance their physical and mental health by including exercise into their daily routine.

A regular schedule can encourage good eating practices, which influence mental health. A balanced diet can assist in controlling mood and energy levels, thereby easing the signs of anxiety and depression. People can make sure they are nourishing their bodies with nutritious foods that support mental wellness by scheduling their meals and snacks as part of their daily routine.

A regular schedule can encourage sound sleep, which is essential for mental wellness. A person can control their sleep habits and make sure they are receiving enough rest by setting a regular bedtime and wake-up time. The ability to regulate mood and lessen the signs of anxiety and depression depends on getting enough sleep.

Creating a daily routine can be a useful strategy for reducing anxiety and depressive symptoms. People can lessen their emotions of anxiety and despair and encourage good behaviors that enhance their mental health by adding structure and predictability to their life.

29 – TREAT UNDERLYING MEDICAL CONDITIONS

Two prevalent mental health issues that can significantly affect a person's life are anxiety and depression. Although while these problems can be treated in a variety of ways, addressing any underlying medical issues can help to reduce symptoms and speed up recovery.

Anxiety and depression may be exacerbated by underlying medical conditions. For instance, anxiety or depression symptoms can be brought on by chronic pain, thyroid issues, or hormonal changes. The symptoms of anxiety and depression can be lessened by treating these underlying illnesses, enabling the patient to feel better and carry out their everyday activities more successfully.

Medication is one of the best approaches to treat underlying medical conditions. For instance, medication can assist in restoring balance and reducing symptoms if a person is experiencing anxiety or depression as a result of an underlying hormonal imbalance. Another example is chronic pain. Taking medication can assist someone suffering from chronic pain to feel less discomfort and in turn ease related symptoms of anxiety and depression.

Additional methods of treating underlying medical issues include dietary and lifestyle modifications, exercise, and stress reduction. Exercise can be especially beneficial in lowering anxiety and depression because it releases endorphins, which enhance mood and lowers stress. Similarly, eating a nutritious diet may contribute to improved physical and mental health while decreasing the likelihood of worsening underlying medical conditions.

Medical treatment may be a necessity for severe cases of anxiety and depression. Your doctor may prescribe anti-anxiety medication and/or antidepressants which may be needed along with counselling and lifestyle modifications (e.g. following the exercises outlined in this book). Some people may be reluctant to start any type of medication. However, getting symptoms under control should be top priority so that time may be invested productively in other areas of our lives rather than spending that same time suffering from anxiety and depression symptoms or even trying to figure out how to resolve them. When the tools are right in front of you, why spend time trying to reinvent the wheel?

Treating underlying medical conditions can be a useful strategy for reducing anxiety and depression. People can lessen their symptoms and enhance their quality of life by addressing any underlying disorders, whether through medication, lifestyle modifications, or other interventions. It is crucial to seek the advice of a healthcare specialist to both investigate potential underlying medical conditions and to provide a suitable treatment regimen.

30 – LIMIT NEGATIVE NEWS OR MEDIA

For people with anxiety and depression, limiting negative news or media may be helpful. Negative thoughts and feelings are a common source of fuel for anxiety and depression, and watching or reading unpleasant news or media can make these feelings worse. Limiting unpleasant news or media might lessen anxiety and depression for the following reasons.

Consuming bad news or media can trigger the sympathetic nervous system, increasing stress hormones like cortisol and adrenaline. The fix is to reduce exposure to negative stimuli. Reducing exposure to stressful situations will lessen the release of stress hormones, which will make people feel calmer and less worried.

Reducing the consumption of unfavorable news and media might encourage optimistic thinking and feelings. When people are not continuously exposed to unpleasant news, they are more inclined to concentrate on the good things that are happening in their life. This can improve their mood and lessen depressive symptoms.

Negative news or media exposure can impair sleep quality, making it challenging for people to get to sleep or stay asleep. Limiting exposure to unfavorable news or media might help improve sleep quality and ease these symptoms because poor sleep can make anxiety and depression symptoms worse.

Reducing unpleasant news or media can help people feel more in control of their environment. Frequent exposure to unfavorable news or media can make people feel helpless and powerless, which can make anxiety and depressive symptoms worse. Regaining control and lessening feelings of helplessness are two benefits of limiting exposure.

Reducing unpleasant news or media might be a useful tactic for treating depression and anxiety. It helps regain control, lessens exposure to stressful stimuli, enhances sleep quality, and enables people to concentrate on the positive elements of their lives.

31 – PRACTICE GRATITUDE

Gratitude exercises are a potent method for reducing anxiety and depression. It is the act of recognizing and appreciating the positive aspects of our lives, both significant and insignificant. This easy technique can help us change our attention from unfavorable to favorable thoughts and reframe our viewpoint to be more favorable.

Negative thoughts and emotions of hopelessness, which can be overpowering and challenging to overcome, frequently drive anxiety and depression. By the practice of thankfulness, we may teach our brains to pay attention to the good things in life even when faced with challenging situations. This mental change can help to give perspective and lessen the intensity of unpleasant feelings.

According to studies, those who regularly express gratitude have lower levels of anxiety and depression. Those who feel grateful are more likely to experience more positive emotions, get better sleep, and have better physical health. In addition to fostering gratitude, resilience and coping mechanisms are also important for overcoming the obstacles life may present.

Keeping a gratitude journal is one way to cultivate gratitude. This entails jotting down each day's blessings, such as a lovely sunset, a thoughtful act from a friend, or just the fact that you have a roof over your head and food on the table. This routine can assist you in refocusing on the positive aspects of your life and cultivating gratitude for the positive aspects that are already there. In more ways than one, the remedy for greed is gratitude.

In general, cultivating gratitude is a straightforward but effective method of lowering anxiety and depression. By concentrating on the positive aspects of our lives, we can develop a sense of perspective and resilience that can make it easier for us to deal with the difficulties of life.

32 – POSITIVE PEOPLE

Anxiety and depression can be significantly reduced by surrounding oneself with positive people. Our mood, conduct, and general mental health can all be impacted by those around us. The optimism, hope, and joy that positive individuals bring into our life can be a potent remedy for unfavorable feelings and thoughts.

We often pick up positive attitudes and habits from the individuals we spend time with. Their upbeat attitude can encourage us, help us feel supported, and make us feel like we belong. As a result of feeling less isolated and more connected to others, anxiety and depressive symptoms can be significantly reduced.

Spending time with negative individuals, though, can have the opposite impact. People with negative attitudes frequently concentrate on issues and challenges, which can lead to a pessimistic outlook and raise tension and worry. Moreover, negative energy can deplete our mental and emotional reserves, leaving us worn out and overburdened.

Consequently, it's essential to surround oneself with uplifting individuals who can aid in our ability to develop resilience, manage stress, and keep a positive outlook. Positive individuals may help us see the good in ourselves and the world around us, as well as challenge us to grow and evolve into better human beings.

The company we keep has a significant influence on our mental health and wellbeing. By giving us a sense of support, optimism, and hope, being around positive people can help us ease anxiety and despair. Making a deliberate effort to find supportive people and form close bonds with them is crucial because doing so can significantly raise our standard of living as a whole.

33 – HOBBIES

A great method to combat anxiety and depression is to take up a hobby. Hobbies provide people with a sense of satisfaction and purpose, which may further improve mood and lower stress levels. Having a pastime can give people a sense of accomplishment and self-worth, which can boost their confidence and self-esteem. Also, hobbies can help people divert their attention away from unfavorable feelings and ideas so that they can concentrate on something fun and good.

Those who enjoy hobbies frequently enter a state of flow in which they are totally absorbed in the action and lose track of time. This can be especially helpful for people who struggle with anxiety or depression because it can make them feel more in the moment and grounded while lowering ruminative thoughts.

Also, hobbies can serve as a social outlet, which can lessen the feelings of loneliness and isolation that frequently go hand in hand with anxiety and depression. When individuals interact via common interests and experiences, participating in a hobby with others can promote a sense of connection and belonging.

Several pastimes, including artistic ones like writing or painting, active ones like yoga or hiking, and social ones like joining a book club or neighborhood sports team, can be helpful for reducing anxiety and depression. A meaningful and gratifying release for stress can be found by discovering a pastime that aligns with one's interests and values.

Taking up a pastime can be a highly effective way to combat anxiety and depression. Hobbies provide people with a sense of success, happiness, and purpose. They also help people concentrate on the here and now and create social ties that can help people feel less alone and isolated.

34 – LEARN A NEW SKILL

One effective strategy to reduce the symptoms of anxiety and depression is by learning a new skill. We can have a sense of mastery and accomplishment that can increase our self-esteem and confidence when we participate in activities that are challenging to us and demand that we learn and improve. This can assist in overcoming the depressive thoughts and hopelessness that frequently accompany anxiety and depression.

A sense of direction and purpose might be one of the main advantages of learning a new skill. Finding motivation or a purpose in life can be challenging when we are dealing with anxiety or depression. Setting and achieving objectives for ourselves can help us develop a sense of direction and focus that can help fight feelings of hopelessness and despair.

Developing a new skill might serve as a beneficial diversion from our anxieties and pessimistic thoughts. We are less prone to dwell on our issues or get into anxious or depressive thought patterns when we are focused on an activity that needs all of our concentration. This might offer a much-needed respite from the incessant mental chatter that can aggravate our discomfort.

Also, developing a new talent can offer a chance for assistance and social interaction. We can meet people who share our passions and interests by enrolling in a class or joining an organization that is linked to our new ability. When someone has anxiety or depression, they frequently experience emotions of loneliness and isolation.

Developing a new talent can be an effective technique for managing anxiety and depression. It can assist in fending off the unfavorable thoughts and sensations that frequently accompany these conditions by giving a sense of purpose, mastery, diversion, and social connection.

35 – HEALTHY THYROID

A tiny, butterfly-shaped gland in the neck called the thyroid is essential for controlling metabolism and creating hormones. Anxiety and depression symptoms might decrease when the thyroid is in good health.

The production of thyroid hormones, particularly triiodothyronine (T3) and thyroxine (T4), by a functioning thyroid is one method that may decrease anxiety and depressive symptoms. The body's metabolism is regulated by these hormones, which in turn influences mood and energy levels. When the thyroid is healthy, it generates enough T3 and T4 to maintain an effective metabolism. This may lead to an increase in energy levels, enhanced concentration and focus, and a better mood.

By the control of serotonin and dopamine levels, the thyroid can also alleviate depression and anxiety. Neurotransmitters like serotonin and dopamine are essential for controlling mood, sleep, hunger, and other biological functions. The production and use of these neurotransmitters can be regulated when the thyroid is operating properly. This may lead to a better mood, less anxiety, and better sleep.

A healthy thyroid can also improve general physical health, which can indirectly promote mental health, in addition to these direct effects on mood and anxiety. For instance, a healthy thyroid can contribute to blood sugar regulation, inflammation reduction, and cardiovascular health. Any of these elements may help you feel better and experience less anxiety and depression.

Maintaining a healthy thyroid is essential for controlling anxiety and depression. A healthy thyroid helps lessen the symptoms of anxiety and depression by creating enough thyroid hormones and controlling neurotransmitters like serotonin and dopamine. A healthy thyroid can also indirectly help to promote mental health by enhancing general physical health.

36 – FORGIVE YOURSELF & OTHERS

Healing emotional scars and getting past unfavorable emotions like anxiety and depression can be accomplished with the help of forgiveness. The act of forgiveness can be transformational, whether it involves forgiving others who have harmed us or forgiving ourselves for past transgressions.

We can get burdened and experience anxiety and sadness when we harbor resentment, rage, or guilt. These unfavorable feelings may prompt us to dwell on the past, which can start a vicious cycle of unfavorable thoughts that can be debilitating. By enabling us to let go of the past and move ahead with a sense of serenity and acceptance, forgiveness ends this cycle.

It might be challenging to forgive someone, especially if they have seriously injured us. However, we only endanger ourselves in the long term by clinging to our wrath and resentment. By making the decision to forgive, we relieve ourselves of the responsibility of clinging to unfavorable feelings and can feel relieved and free.

Along with forgiving others, it's equally important to forgive oneself. We are frequently the toughest judges of ourselves, and self-blame can be a major factor in anxiety and depression. We can raise our self-esteem and lessen critical self-talk by forgiving ourselves for our previous transgressions and letting go of self-judgment.

Forgiving someone takes time and work, but it is well worth the effort.

By forgiving others, we can overcome the unfavorable feelings that fuel anxiety and depression and enjoy higher emotional wellbeing and happiness.

37 – AVOID ISOLATION

Humans need to interact with others on a basic level. Isolating oneself may have a significant negative effect on mental health, increasing levels of anxiety and depression.

A couple of the most prevalent mental health conditions worldwide are anxiety and depression. Numerous things, including genetics, life events, and environmental factors, can contribute to their development. The development and aggravation of these illnesses, however, can also be significantly influenced by social isolation.

People who are isolated may experience feelings of loneliness, disconnection, and unsupportiveness. These emotions can induce a sensation of helplessness and despair, setting off a chain reaction of unfavorable feelings. Maintaining social relationships, on the other hand, can encourage feelings of happiness, belonging, and purpose, which can assist to fight sadness and anxiety.

Social support can significantly affect mental health, according to studies. People who are socially connected have lower rates of anxiety and depression than people who are socially isolated. Social connections provide a sense of belonging, practical support, and emotional support, all of which can help to lower stress and enhance mental health.

Social connection can also give people a sense of direction and meaning. Volunteering, taking part in hobbies and interests with others, and participating in social events can all lead to a higher sense of fulfillment and enjoyment, which helps lessen anxiety and depression.

Preventing and decreasing anxiety and depression requires taking steps to avoid isolation. People can reap the various advantages of social support, such as emotional support, practical aid, a sense of belonging and purpose, by maintaining social relationships. Making social relationships a priority can help people live happier and more meaningful lives by enhancing their mental health.

38 – SET BOUNDARIES

For the sake of maintaining good relationships and practicing self-care, limits must be set. Boundaries are restrictions that people set for themselves in order to maintain their physical, emotional, and mental health. Boundaries are important to establish and uphold because they greatly reduce anxiety and depression.

A common cause of anxiety and depression is a sense of helplessness or being overwhelmed. Setting boundaries enables people to take charge of their lives and cultivate a sense of empowerment. By making people feel more in control of their lives and their relationships, this can lessen feelings of anxiety and depression. Setting limits in a love relationship, for instance, might help people avoid becoming overtaken or exhausted by their partner's emotional needs.

Establishing boundaries encourages self-care, which is crucial for maintaining mental health. Setting boundaries allows people to put their own needs and wellbeing first, which can lessen stress and anxiety. Saying "no" to extra duties at work or home or taking time for oneself to recharge are both effective ways to do this.

Setting limits can also help relationships by enhancing communication and lowering conflict. People lessen the possibility of misunderstandings and resentment when they explain their limits in a clear and aggressive manner. This can lessen the anxiety and depressive symptoms that result from stressful relationships.

By encouraging a sense of control, lowering stress and conflict in relationships, and encouraging self-care, setting boundaries can lessen anxiety and depression. To preserve healthy relationships and well-being, it is imperative to recognize one's own boundaries and express them firmly.

39 – LEARN TO SAY NO

Saying no is a crucial ability that can significantly improve our mental health. Saying yes to everything often results in us taking on more than we can handle. This can be especially difficult for people who struggle with anxiety and depression because the added demands may not only be overwhelming and stressful but may also worsen the symptoms.

Learning to say no allows us to prioritize our own needs and well-being, which is one of the main advantages. We may free up time and energy to concentrate on the things that mean most to us when we learn to say no to things that are not necessary or do not reflect our beliefs. This might help us feel like we have greater control over our life and can lessen stress and worry.

We can establish boundaries and effectively express our needs by saying no. For those who struggle with self-advocacy and assertiveness due to anxiety or depression, this can be especially crucial. We may develop our self-assurance and assert ourselves in a way that seems genuine and courteous by learning to say no.

Saying no also has the potential to lessen feelings of shame and guilt. Saying yes to things we don't want to do can make us feel resentful and bitter, which can result in self-talk that is critical of ourselves and self-blame. By refusing, we can steer clear of these unpleasant feelings and put our attention on the things that make us happy and fulfilled.

Developing the ability to say no is a crucial skill that can significantly affect our mental health. We can decrease stress, prevent being overwhelmed, boost our confidence and self-esteem, and cultivate a greater sense of control and well-being in our lives by setting boundaries, prioritizing our needs, and communicating clearly.

40 – MEDITATE

For centuries, people have practiced meditation to enhance both their mental and physical well-being. It is now widely acknowledged as a useful technique for controlling anxiety and depression. Millions of people worldwide are afflicted by the prevalent mental health diseases of anxiety and depression. They can significantly impact our daily activities, such as work, school, and social life. Meditation has been proven to help with relieving the symptoms of anxiety and depression and enhancing our general wellbeing.

By creating inner peace and tranquility and soothing the mind, meditation has a calming effect. When we meditate, we concentrate on the here and now, which enables us to let go of problems and unfavorable ideas. This promotes relaxation and lowers stress levels, which can be very helpful for people with anxiety and depression. In fact, studies have shown that regular meditation can cut down on the signs of depression and anxiety by as much as 50%.

Regulating the autonomic nerve system is one of the main ways meditation reduces anxiety and sadness. This area of the nervous system regulates how the body reacts to stress. The "fight or flight" reaction, which can cause a variety of physical and mental symptoms, including a rapid heartbeat, shallow breathing, and feelings of panic, is triggered by stress or worry, and is controlled by the autonomic nervous system. The relaxation response, which balances the stress response and lessens the symptoms of anxiety and depression, can be triggered by meditation.

A fundamental component of controlling anxiety and depression is emotional regulation, which can be improved by meditation. Regular meditation practice can help us become more self-aware and in control by teaching us how to notice our thoughts and emotions without passing judgment. By doing so, we can lessen the strength and frequency of unpleasant feelings while also being able to react to stressful events more effectively.

A simple way to start meditating is by either sitting on the floor or in a chair with your spine straight and eyes closed. For beginners, set your phone timer for two minutes. Sit straight, relax, and take deep breaths – inhale, exhale. All you should be focusing on and doing for two minutes is your breathing. As you get better, gradually increase the time. Once again, practice makes perfect.

Meditation is an effective method for controlling anxiety and depression and may help people feel more at ease, in control of their lives, and relaxed by encouraging relaxation, controlling the autonomic nervous system, and enhancing emotional regulation. With consistent practice, meditation may be a vital tool to help facilitate mental health and wellbeing.

41 – PRAY

A higher power, such as God, the universe, or any other spiritual force, can be reached by praying. It is a custom shared by many faiths and is frequently employed as a means of consolation, direction, and support. There are many mental health advantages of praying, including a reduction in anxiety and depression and most important of all, hope.

Praying serves to foster a sense of tranquility and relaxation, which is one of the key reasons it can reduce anxiety and depression. People frequently let go of their problems and stressors when praying and concentrate on their breathing. This can aid in easing stress and fostering a sense of tranquility and harmony. Additionally, praying can heighten feelings of hope and optimism, which can balance out the unfavorable feelings and thoughts that frequently go along with anxiety and depression.

Prayer can foster a sense of community and connection. Many people take solace in the idea that they are not alone and that there is a greater power who hears their prayers and provides them with assistance and advice. Feelings of loneliness and isolation, which are common risk factors for anxiety and depression, can be lessened by doing this.

By encouraging a sense of thankfulness and appreciation, prayer can also help with anxiety and despair. Regular prayers frequently express thankfulness for their blessings, including their health, loved ones, and friends. Putting more emphasis on these positive facets of life can help to divert attention from unfavorable feelings and thoughts and encourage a more upbeat outlook.

As a result, praying may be a useful strategy for lowering anxiety and depression. It offers a sense of serenity, hope, community, and thankfulness. Consider including prayer in your daily routine if you experience anxiety or depression to see how it might provide you comfort and vigor.

42 – LAUGH

Laughing is an effective therapy for easing anxiety and depression. It sets off a variety of physiological and psychological reactions that can be beneficial to our mental and emotional well-being. Our bodies produce endorphins when we laugh, which are organic mood enhancers that can lessen stress and anxiety. Moreover, endorphins enhance happiness, which might lessen the effects of depression.

Laughter not only releases endorphins but also lowers cortisol levels, a stress hormone that, when persistently raised, can have several detrimental impacts on health. As laughter lowers cortisol levels, it can aid in promoting relaxation and easing anxiety symptoms.

Laughing can enhance our outlook on life as a whole. When we laugh, we change our attention from unfavorable feelings and thoughts to the good things in life. This can help us feel better and lessen the effects of depression. Laughing can strengthen our bonds with others and lessen feelings of loneliness or isolation, which can exacerbate anxiety and depression.

In general, laughter is a highly effective technique to combat anxiety and depression. It causes a variety of physiological and psychological reactions that can improve our mental health. Thus, if you're feeling nervous or depressed, try watching a comedy (you can find hundreds of stand-up comedians and sitcoms on YouTube for free), hanging out with funny people, or even doing some laughter yoga - you might find that it significantly improves your mood and mental health.

43 – PHYSICAL ACTIVITY

Exercise has been shown to be a successful treatment for depression and anxiety symptoms. Endorphins are naturally occurring substances that cause sensations of happiness and well-being and are released during exercise. Moreover, regular exercise can aid in lowering cortisol levels, a hormone linked to stress and anxiety.

Physical activity helps to boost feelings of positivity and self-confidence by diverting attention from negative thoughts and worries. Exercise also fosters a sense of achievement, which can enhance mood and lessen worry.

Exercise has been found in studies to be just as effective as medicine in the treatment of mild to moderate depression and anxiety. In fact, it has been discovered that regular exercise is more effective than medication at preventing depressive relapses.

Engaging in physical activity fosters a sense of social connection, which is advantageous for people who are dealing with depression or anxiety. A sense of support and community can be created by joining a sports team or group fitness class, which can help fight feelings of loneliness.

Exercise can enhance the quality of sleep, which is crucial for general mental health. Mood regulation and anxiety reduction depend on getting enough sleep.

Engaging in physical activity can help reduce the effects of anxiety and depression. It can enhance general mental health and wellbeing and is a natural, inexpensive therapeutic option. A better, healthier life can result from including regular exercise in one's everyday routine.

44 – COMFORT ZONE

Two of the most prevalent mental health conditions that affect people of all ages, races, and socioeconomic backgrounds are anxiety and depression. The propensity to stick to one's comfort zone is one of the many diverse causes of these diseases. The psychological state in which a person feels at ease, secure, and at home is known as the comfort zone. It is a place where one can stay away from dangers and difficulties that might make them feel uneasy or anxious.

But according to studies, adhering to one's comfort zone may actually make anxiety and depression worse. Avoiding risks and challenges might cause people to lose out on significant chances for progress. Moreover, avoiding obstacles might result in a sensation of stagnation and monotony.

By stepping out of one's comfort zone, you expose yourself to more opportunities to succeed in life. People can learn new abilities and skills when they push themselves and engage in novel experiences. Increased confidence, self-esteem, and a sense of success can result from this, which helps lessen depressive and anxious sensations.

Some simple examples of stepping out of your comfort zone are as follows.

1. Go to the library instead of reading at home
2. Go to the gym instead of working out at home
3. Go outside for a walk instead of using a treadmill

4. Go out shopping instead of ordering online
5. Cook instead of eating fast food

It's important to step out of our comfort zone intermittently to expose yourself to challenges and what may seem difficult and to perhaps find more windows of opportunity.

Setting small, doable goals is one approach to leaving your comfort zone. For instance, if you're afraid of speaking in front of large groups, you might start by doing so in small groups. You may progressively increase the audience size as you get more at ease with it until you feel comfortable speaking in front of sizable crowds.

Setting objectives and getting assistance can both be beneficial. As you attempt to venture outside of your comfort zone, joining a support group, consulting a therapist, or confiding in a close friend can offer encouragement and accountability.

Stepping outside of your comfort zone can help to reduce anxiety and depression. You may learn new talents and boost your confidence by pushing yourself and doing new things, which will make your life feel more fulfilling and satisfying. More importantly, you will be better prepared and well equipped when life forces you to step out of your comfort zone.

45 – RESPECT YOURSELF

Respecting yourself is crucial to keeping your mental health in check and may be quite helpful in reducing anxiety and depression. Respecting yourself makes it more likely that you will prioritize self-care, establish healthy boundaries, and engage in behaviors and relationships that are consistent with your values and objectives.

When we ignore our own needs and desires, we nurture anxiety and depression, creating a sense of alienation and discontent with our lives. This might make us feel overburdened, powerless, and hopeless, which can make anxiety and depressive symptoms worse.

You are proactive by treating yourself with respect. For instance, taking care of your physical and mental health by getting enough sleep, eating well, and exercising frequently will help to lessen the symptoms of depression and anxiety.

By providing you greater control over your time and energy, setting good boundaries and even learning to say no can aid in the reduction of stress and anxiety. You are prioritizing your own needs and decreasing the possibility of burnout and overwhelm when you respect yourself enough to say no to activities or relationships that exhaust you.

Finally, pursuing relationships and activities that are consistent with your beliefs and objectives can help you feel fulfilled and purposeful, which can lessen feelings of hopelessness and sadness. You are more likely to experience a sense of purpose and fulfillment in life when you respect yourself enough to go for the things that are actually important to you.

Overall, having self-respect is crucial to sustaining mental health, and it can significantly help with the symptoms of anxiety and depression. You may enhance your general well-being and lessen symptoms of stress, anxiety, and depression by prioritizing self-care, establishing appropriate boundaries, and engaging in meaningful activities and relationships.

46 – EDUCATE YOURSELF

A helpful method of battling depression and anxiety is education. People might feel more in charge of their mental health and lessen their symptoms by becoming educated about the illnesses, their causes, and potential solutions.

Understanding anxiety and depression can help people relate to their feelings and lessen the stigma associated with these diseases. Individuals might identify that their experiences are not unique or humiliating, but rather normal and treatable, by learning about the typical symptoms, causes, and therapies. Knowing this can assist in lessening the emotions of loneliness and guilt that are frequently accompanied with anxiety and depression.

Education can assist people in recognizing successful coping mechanisms and available therapies. People can create a unique plan for controlling their symptoms by learning about the advantages of exercise, mindfulness, and cognitive-behavioral therapy, for instance. Also, being aware of the advantages and disadvantages of a medicine can help a person choose their course of therapy with knowledge.

Education may give people a sense of direction and significance. People can gain a sense of success and self-esteem by seeking information and picking up new abilities, which can be beneficial for mental health. Also, by learning about issues that interest them, people can find a purpose in their lives and become more motivated, which can help them fight the feelings of hopelessness and apathy that are frequently connected with anxiety and depression.

Learning more about anxiety and depression can be a very effective management strategy. People can take control of their mental health and enhance their general wellbeing by minimizing stigma, identifying helpful coping mechanisms and treatment alternatives, and generating a sense of purpose and meaning.

47 - DELAYED GRATIFICATION

The act of delaying immediate benefits or pleasure in favor of a more important, long-term advantage is referred to as delayed gratification. Delaying gratification is a crucial skill for emotional control and mental health, according to research. Delaying pleasure in particular helps lessen the signs of anxiety and depression.

Millions of people worldwide are afflicted by the complicated mental health diseases of anxiety and depression. While depression is defined by continuous sadness and a sense of helplessness, anxiety is characterized by excessive concern and fear. Both disorders have the potential to significantly impede daily functioning and lower a person's quality of life.

One of the ways delayed gratification reduces anxiety and depression is by enhancing one's capacity for self-control and self-discipline. Delaying gratification gives people the power and assurance that they can control their desires and make wise judgments. This might lessen hopelessness and feelings of helplessness that frequently accompany depression and anxiety.

Delaying pleasure can also give people a sense of direction and purpose. Long-term goals provide people with a sense of purpose and fulfillment that might help them cope with negative emotions. This sense of direction can aid people in adopting a more upbeat attitude on life and boosting their overall resilience.

Instant gratification is the opposite of delayed gratification and refers to the temptation to choose immediate pleasure over future benefit.

Delaying gratification allows people to concentrate on the here and now, which lowers stress and anxiety. Those who practice delayed gratification are more likely to concentrate on the procedures necessary to reach their objectives rather than being preoccupied by immediate desires. This can aid people in becoming more focused and present, which can lessen depressive and anxious symptoms.

48 – AVOID NEGATIVE PEOPLE

It's a widely accepted concept that we are comprised of the individuals we spend the most time with. Spending time with upbeat, inspiring people tends to make us feel better about ourselves and our life. On the other hand, if we are surrounded by negative people, we could experience anxiety, depression, and exhaustion.

It's possible to reduce anxiety and depression by avoiding unpleasant people. Spending time with people who are continuously critical and negative might cause us to internalize their negativity, which can cause us to experience feelings of hopelessness and despair. Our mental health could be affected if we start to doubt our own worth and ability.

Negative people frequently add drama and disorder to our lives, too. They could cause unneeded stress, spread stories or gossip, and overall put us on edge. For those who already experience anxiety or depression, this could be very harmful.

Spending time with upbeat, encouraging people, on the other hand, can have the opposite impact. These people might serve as a source of motivation and inspiration, assisting us in seeing the best in both us and the world around us. They might provide us with sound guidance and a sympathetic ear, establishing a secure environment in which we can explore our emotions and ideas.

It's crucial to understand that avoiding unfavorable people doesn't necessarily entail excluding them from our life completely. Setting boundaries and limiting our exposure to negativity may be all we need to do at times. By doing this, we may cultivate an environment that is more encouraging and supportive for ourselves, which can have a significant effect on our mental health and general welfare.

49 – TIME MANAGEMENT

One's mental health can be greatly impacted by having effective time management skills. Two of the most prevalent mental health conditions are anxiety and depression, both of which can become worse over time if there is a lack of control. People may experience anxiety and depression when they feel overburdened by their obligations and don't have a clear strategy for managing their time.

By giving one's daily life structure and organization, effective time management can aid in reducing negative sensations. People can feel more in control of their time and experience less stress and anxiety by making a schedule and prioritizing their responsibilities. Those who have a strategy in place are less likely to feel overburdened by their obligations and are better able to approach each activity with clarity and purpose.

In addition, time management can aid in lowering the risk of procrastination, which is a frequent source of stress and anxiety. Those who procrastinate may feel guilty or ashamed, which might result in unhappy thoughts and depressive sensations. Individuals are more likely to stay on task and refrain from procrastinating when they have a defined strategy for managing their time.

Effective time management can also result in more production, which raises one's self-esteem and lessens depressive symptoms. People feel a sense of pleasure and success when they are able to complete their tasks and meet their deadlines, which can elevate their mood and overall mental health.

Time management is an effective technique that helps lessen depression and anxiety. People can feel more in control of their time, have less stress and anxiety, be more productive, and have higher self-esteem by adding structure and organization to their lives.

50 – ANGER MANAGEMENT

It's not unusual for someone with anger issues to simultaneously struggle with anxiety and depression. Rage and anxiety frequently go hand in hand. Extreme anger causes the body to release adrenaline, which can result in physical symptoms including accelerated heartbeat, perspiration, and even panic attacks. This ongoing tension can eventually cause anxiety and depression.

The physical signs of anger can be controlled, and rage outbursts can be less frequent and intense by using anger management practices. The underlying emotional and psychological problems that cause anger, anxiety, and sadness may also benefit from these treatments.

Cognitive behavioral therapy is a powerful method for controlling anger (CBT). CBT enables people to recognize and alter harmful thought patterns that fuel rage and anxiety. Anger and anxiety can be reduced by teaching oneself to replace negative thoughts with positive ones.

Another method for controlling rage, anxiety, and sadness is mindfulness meditation. Focusing on the present moment while accepting one's thoughts and feelings without judgment is the goal of mindfulness meditation. This can assist people in developing better emotional regulation and awareness of their anger triggers.

Exercising regularly can help you control your anger, anxiety, and depression. Workout releases natural mood enhancers called endorphins. Moreover, regular exercise can raise emotions of wellbeing, enhance sleep, and lessen feelings of tension and worry.

Anger management can be a useful tool for lowering the risk of anxiety and depression. People can enhance their overall quality of life and lessen the damaging effects that prolonged stress can have on their mental and physical health by learning how to control their anger in a healthy way.

CONCLUSION

In conclusion, there are numerous efficient strategies to treat anxiety and depression. As mentioned in the introduction of this book, anxiety and depression don't come knocking and when they arrive it's best to be prepared. Having the tools beforehand speeds up the process of recovery and prevention. As outlined in this book, there are several methods that people can take to enhance their mental health and well-being, including physical activities like walking and strength training, mindfulness techniques like meditation and deep breathing, social relationships, and getting professional treatment in the form of medication and counselling. It's crucial to keep in mind that everyone's path to better mental health is different, and it's okay to explore various strategies before settling on one that works best for you. Anxiety and depression can be managed and even beaten with time, self-compassion, and support from loved ones. Always keep in mind that asking for assistance is a sign of strength, and there is always hope for a better tomorrow.

ABOUT THE AUTHOR

Dr. R. Ahmed is all about improving quality of life. Through his many roles in life, he has frequently engaged in the art of leveraging by:

- Leveraging Medicine and Counseling to manage mental health (as a Physician)
- Leveraging Medicine, Education, and Lifestyle modifications to both cure and prevent disease (as a Physician)
- Leveraging Technology to improve patient care (as an Engineer)
- Leveraging Technology to improve investing strategies (as an Investor)
- Leveraging Education to help find jobs in Healthcare Informatics (as a Professor)
- Leveraging Sports and Academics to improve life (as a Mentor, Coach, and Teacher)
- Leveraging Books to improve quality of life (as an Author)

Don't forget to leave a review and please visit our website: BOOKPASSION.NET

Thank you!

Printed in Great Britain
by Amazon